LOW PURINE DIET PLAN COOK BOOK

The Complete Low Purine Diet Plan: Nutritious Culinary Practices for Managing Uric Acid Levels

REX LEWIS

Table of Contents

Introduction

Purines are essential chemical substances involved in the composition of DNA and RNA, which are the genetic material found in all living cells. Nitrogen-containing compounds that act as the foundation for nucleic acid synthesis. There are two primary types of purines: adenine and guanine. Purines are necessary for cell function, but their metabolism can impact health, especially in situations like gout.

Key Elements to Comprehend About Purines and Their Influence On Health:

Role in DNA and RNA:

• Adenine and guanine, the two types of purines, are fundamental components of DNA and RNA. They form base pairs with specific pyrimidines (thymine in DNA, uracil in RNA, and cytosine in both), contributing to the structure and function of these genetic materials.

Purine Metabolism:

• Purines can be derived from the diet or synthesized within the body. The breakdown of purines results in the formation of uric acid.

Uric Acid and Health:

• Uric acid is the end product of purine metabolism. It is typically excreted through the kidneys. Elevated levels of uric acid in the blood can lead to health issues, particularly gout.

Gout:

• Gout is a type of arthritis caused by the deposition of urate crystals in joints and tissues. Excessive consumption of purine-rich foods, along with impaired excretion of uric acid, can contribute to the development of gout.

Purine-Rich Foods:

• Foods high in purines include organ meats (liver, kidney), certain seafood (anchovies, sardines, mussels), red meat, and some alcoholic beverages (beer). Limiting the intake of these foods is often recommended for individuals with gout or those at risk.

Individual Variability:

• The impact of purines on health can vary from person to person. Some individuals may be more susceptible to gout or may have conditions affecting purine metabolism.

Balanced Diet:

• It's important to maintain a balanced diet that includes a variety of foods. While certain purine-rich foods should be consumed in moderation, other dietary and lifestyle factors also play a role in overall health.

Medical Conditions:

• Certain medical conditions and medications can influence purine metabolism. Individuals with conditions such as kidney disease or those taking medications that affect uric acid levels should be monitored by healthcare professionals.

Purines are crucial for life, but their metabolism and consequent uric acid levels must be carefully controlled to avoid health problems like gout. It is crucial to maintain a balanced diet, stay hydrated, and consult a doctor if there are concerns about uric acid levels to manage purine-related health problems.

CHAPTER ONE
Purine-Rich Foods

Purine-rich foods are those with elevated purine levels that can be converted into uric acid in the body. It is advisable for patients with gout or those aiming to control uric acid levels to restrict their consumption of certain foods. Not all purine-rich foods must be entirely avoided; moderation is essential. Here are some examples of foods high in purines:

Organ Meats:

- Liver
- Kidneys
- Heart
- Sweetbreads

Seafood:

- Anchovies
- Sardines
- Mussels
- Herring
- Trout
- Mackerel

Game Meats:

- Venison
- Game birds (e.g., pheasant, duck)

Red Meat:

- Beef
- Pork
- Lamb

Processed Meats:

- Bacon

- Sausages

- Hot dogs

Gravy and Broths:

- Gravies made from meat drippings

- Organ meat broths

Yeast Extracts:

- Yeast extract spreads

- Brewer's yeast

- Certain Vegetables:

- Asparagus

- Spinach (contains moderately high levels)

Alcoholic Beverages:

- Beer, especially certain types with higher yeast content
- Some types of spirits

Not all purine-rich foods must be completely removed from the diet; many can be consumed in moderation. Dietary choices are just one component of a healthy lifestyle. Hydration, weight management, and regular exercise are also crucial variables in controlling uric acid levels.

Individuals with concerns about gout or excessive uric acid levels should seek individualized counsel from a healthcare expert or a trained dietitian due to potential variations in responses to purine-rich meals.

Health Conditions and Purine Levels

The significance of purine levels on health is especially important in relation to specific medical diseases, with gout being the most prominent example. Gout is a form of arthritis distinguished by the accumulation of urate crystals in joints, resulting in inflammation and discomfort. Increased uric acid levels in the bloodstream, caused by the breakdown of purines, lead to the onset of gout. It's important to note that elevated uric acid levels do not guarantee the development of gout, as other variables can contribute to the condition.

Here are some health conditions and factors related to purine levels:

Gout:

• Gout is linked to high levels of uric acid, which can be caused by consuming purine-rich meals, reduced uric acid excretion, or a combination of both factors. Management typically requires dietary adjustments, lifestyle alterations, and occasionally medication..

Kidney Stones:

• Elevated uric acid levels can lead to the development of kidney stones, especially if urate crystals build up in the kidneys. People who have had kidney stones in the past should keep track of how much purine they consume.

Kidney Disease:

• Conditions that damage the kidneys, like chronic renal disease, can reduce the body's efficiency in excreting uric acid. This can result in elevated amounts of uric acid in the bloodstream.

Hypertension (High Blood Pressure):

• Some research indicates a possible connection between high levels of uric acid and hypertension. The relationship is intricate and not completely comprehended.

Metabolic Syndrome:

• Metabolic syndrome is a collection of illnesses such as abdominal obesity, hypertension, hyperglycemia, and abnormal lipid profiles. Research indicates a correlation between metabolic syndrome and increased uric acid levels.

Certain Medications:

• Some medications, such as diuretics (water pills) and certain immunosuppressive drugs, can impact uric acid levels. It's important for individuals on these medications to be monitored by healthcare professionals.

It is essential to address the connection between purines and health with subtlety. High purine intake can increase uric acid levels, although genetics, general diet, and lifestyle also influence these situations. It is advisable for those worried about health problems associated to purine to get advice from a healthcare professional or a trained dietician. They can offer customized guidance according to the person's health condition and assist in creating a strategy that harmonizes food selections with general health requirements.

CHAPTER TWO
Benefits of a Low Purine Diet

A reduced purine diet can be advantageous for persons with specific health concerns including gout, kidney stones, or kidney disease. Below are some possible advantages linked to following a low purine diet:

• Decreased likelihood of Gout Attacks: Gout is a kind of arthritis resulting from the accumulation of urate crystals in the joints, causing inflammation and discomfort. Restricting purine consumption can lower uric acid production in patients with gout, potentially reducing the risk of gout attacks.

- A reduced purine diet can help reduce uric acid levels in the bloodstream. It is crucial for persons predisposed to hyperuricemia, which is associated with gout and other related disorders.

- **Prevention of Kidney Stones:** - Elevated levels of uric acid in the urine might lead to the development of kidney stones. Regulating purine consumption can help lower the likelihood of developing uric acid kidney stones.

- **Enhanced renal Function:** A low purine diet can be advantageous for persons with renal disease, especially those with impaired kidney function. The kidneys excrete uric acid, therefore lowering dietary purines can help lessen the workload on the kidneys.

- **Management of Comorbid Health Conditions:** Research indicates possible connections between increased uric acid levels and health issues such as hypertension and metabolic syndrome. Following a reduced purine diet can benefit cardiovascular health and metabolic wellness.

- **Weight Management:** Some high-purine foods, like red meat and processed meats, are linked to increased calorie and fat levels. Opting for a reduced purine diet can indirectly aid in weight control and encourage a healthier body weight.

- **Improved Joint Health:** Reducing purine-rich foods can help alleviate inflammation in patients with inflammatory joint diseases, while the main association with joint health is shown in gout.

A reduced purine diet should be followed with attention to maintaining balance and considering overall nutritional requirements. It is important to prioritize essential nutrients and seek tailored advice from healthcare specialists or registered dietitians. Hydration, dietary patterns, and lifestyle choices are important elements that contribute significantly to supporting overall health in addition to managing purine consumption.

Planning a Low Purine Diet

Creating a low purine diet requires careful selection of items to reduce purine consumption. This can be especially advantageous for patients with illnesses like gout, kidney stones, or kidney disease. Here are some basic principles to assist in creating a reduced purine diet plan:

Focus on Low-Purine Foods:

Choose foods that are low in purines, including:

- Fruits (except certain high-purine fruits like cherries and bananas, which should be consumed in moderation)

- Vegetables (except asparagus and spinach, which have moderate purine content)

Whole grains

- Low-fat or fat-free dairy products
- Eggs
- Nuts and seeds in moderation

Limit High-Purine Foods:

Reduce or avoid foods high in purines, including:

- Organ meats (liver, kidney, sweetbreads)

- Certain seafood (anchovies, sardines, mussels, herring)
- Red meat (beef, pork, lamb)
- Game meats
- Processed meats (bacon, sausages, hot dogs)
- Gravy and organ meat broths
- Yeast extracts (e.g., spreads, brewer's yeast)

Choose Lean Protein Sources:

Opt for lean sources of protein, such as poultry, fish (except high-purine varieties), tofu, and legumes. These can provide adequate protein without significantly increasing purine intake.

Stay Hydrated: Adequate hydration helps flush out uric acid from the body. Drinking plenty of water is important for overall health and can be beneficial for individuals on a low purine diet.

Moderate Alcohol Consumption:

• Limit or avoid alcohol, especially beer, as it is associated with higher purine content. Moderate consumption of wine or spirits may be acceptable for some individuals, but it's essential to consult with a healthcare professional.

Monitor Portion Sizes: Controlling portion sizes can help manage overall purine intake. Smaller portions of high-purine foods may be included occasionally, but moderation is key.

Choose Low-Fat Options: Opt for low-fat or fat-free dairy products and lean cuts of meat. This not only helps manage purine intake but also supports overall heart health.

Consider Personalized Recommendations: Individuals may have different tolerances to purines, and personalized recommendations from a healthcare professional or registered dietitian can provide tailored guidance based on specific health conditions, medications, and dietary preferences.

Ensure that a low purine diet maintains overall nutritional balance. It is crucial to uphold a balanced diet that consists of a diverse range of nutrient-dense foods. For tailored guidance about health issues associated to purine metabolism, it is recommended to seek advice from a healthcare expert or a qualified dietitian.

CHAPTER THREE

Low Purine Diet Recipes

Developing low purine diet recipes requires choosing items that are low in purines yet still offer tasty and nourishing meals. Here are some suggestions for recipes low in purine content:

1. Grilled Lemon Herb Chicken

Ingredients:

- Skinless, boneless chicken breasts
- Fresh lemon juice
- Olive oil
- Garlic (minced)
- Fresh herbs (such as rosemary, thyme, or parsley)

- Salt and pepper to taste

Instructions:

1. Combine lemon juice, olive oil, minced garlic, chopped herbs, salt, and pepper in a basin to make a marinade.

2. Allow the chicken breasts to marinate in the sauce for a minimum of 30 minutes.

3. Preheat the grill and cook the chicken thoroughly, flipping it occasionally.

4. Accompany with steamed veggies or a green salad.

2. Quinoa and Vegetable Stir-Fry

Ingredients:

- Quinoa
- Mixed vegetables (bell peppers, zucchini, broccoli, carrots)
- Low-sodium soy sauce
- Garlic (minced)
- Ginger (grated)
- Sesame oil
- Scallions (chopped)

Instructions:

1. Cook quinoa according to package instructions.
2. In a pan, sauté minced garlic and grated ginger in sesame oil.
3. Add mixed vegetables and stir-fry until tender-crisp.

4. Toss in cooked quinoa and drizzle with low-sodium soy sauce.

5. Garnish with chopped scallions before serving.

3. Baked Salmon with Dill Sauce

Ingredients:

- Salmon fillets
- Fresh dill (chopped)
- Lemon slices
- Greek yogurt
- Dijon mustard
- Salt and pepper to taste

Instructions:

1. Preheat the oven and place salmon fillets on a baking sheet.

2. Season with salt, pepper, and chopped dill.

3. Top each fillet with a lemon slice and bake until the salmon is cooked through.

4. In a bowl, mix Greek yogurt, Dijon mustard, and more fresh dill to create a sauce.

5. Serve the baked salmon with the dill sauce on the side.

4. Lentil and Vegetable Soup

Ingredients:

- Lentils
- Mixed vegetables (carrots, celery, onions)
- Low-sodium vegetable broth
- Garlic (minced)

- Cumin and coriander (ground)

- Fresh parsley (chopped)

- Salt and pepper to taste

Instructions:

1. In a pot, sauté minced garlic in olive oil until fragrant.

2. Add mixed vegetables and cook until softened.

3. Stir in lentils, ground cumin, and coriander.

4. Pour in low-sodium vegetable broth and simmer until lentils are tender.

5. Season with salt, pepper, and garnish with fresh parsley before serving.

These recipes provide tasty and fulfilling choices for a low-purine diet. Customize recipes to suit individual tastes and dietary requirements, and seek guidance from a healthcare provider or qualified dietitian for specific recommendations.

Lifestyle Changes for Managing Purine Levels

Regulating purine levels requires implementing dietary adjustments and incorporating specific lifestyle changes to enhance general well-being. Here are some lifestyle modifications that can assist in controlling purine levels:

Hydration:

• Adequate hydration is crucial for flushing out uric acid from the body. Drink plenty of water throughout the day to help maintain good kidney function and prevent the crystallization of urate in the joints.

Maintain a Healthy Weight:

• Obesity is a risk factor for gout and other metabolic conditions. Losing excess weight can contribute to the reduction of uric acid levels. Adopting a balanced diet and engaging in regular physical activity can support weight management.

Regular Exercise:

• Regular physical activity has multiple benefits, including weight management and improved overall health. Exercise can also help regulate insulin levels, which may indirectly influence uric acid metabolism. Consult with a healthcare professional before starting a new exercise routine, especially if there are existing health conditions.

Limit Alcohol Consumption:

• Alcohol, particularly beer, has been associated with elevated uric acid levels. Limiting or avoiding alcohol, especially for individuals with gout or a predisposition to hyperuricemia, can be beneficial.

Limit Sugar-Sweetened Beverages:

• High fructose intake, often found in sugar-sweetened beverages, has been linked to increased uric acid levels. Reducing the consumption of these beverages can be helpful.

Moderate Protein Intake:

• While some proteins are high in purines, it's important to maintain a balanced protein intake. Opt for lean protein sources such as poultry, fish, tofu, and legumes.

Stress Management:

• Chronic stress can contribute to various health issues, including inflammatory conditions. Implement stress-reducing techniques such as mindfulness, meditation, or yoga to support overall well-being.

Adequate Sleep:

• Poor sleep has been associated with various health problems, including metabolic disturbances. Aim for 7-9 hours of quality sleep per night to support overall health.

Regular Health Check-ups:

• Regular monitoring of uric acid levels and overall health through routine check-ups is essential. This allows for early detection of any issues and adjustments to the management plan as needed.

Medication Adherence:

• If prescribed medication to manage uric acid levels, it's crucial to adhere to the prescribed treatment plan. Regular follow-ups with healthcare professionals can help ensure the effectiveness of the medication.

It is important to make lifestyle modifications with the guidance of healthcare specialists, particularly for persons with pre-existing health concerns. An integrated strategy incorporating dietary adjustments, lifestyle alterations, and suitable medical treatment can effectively control purine levels and associated health issues.

Supplements and Medications

Supplements and drugs may be included in the treatment regimen for persons with illnesses associated with purine levels, including gout or hyperuricemia. Consult a healthcare expert before using supplements or drugs to receive individualized advice based on unique health needs. Below are typical vitamins and drugs utilized in treating purine-related conditions:

Medications:

Urate-Lowering Drugs:

• **Allopurinol:** This medication inhibits the enzyme responsible for the production of uric acid. It is often prescribed for individuals with gout or those with recurrent kidney stones.

• **Febuxostat:** Similar to allopurinol, febuxostat reduces uric acid production and is used in the management of gout.

Prophylaxis for Gout Attacks:

• **Colchicine:** This medication helps reduce inflammation and pain associated with gout attacks. It is sometimes used prophylactically during the initiation of urate-lowering therapy.

Anti-Inflammatory Drugs:

• **Nonsteroidal Anti-Inflammatory Drugs (NSAIDs):** These drugs, such as ibuprofen or naproxen, can help manage pain and inflammation during gout attacks.

• **Corticosteroids:** In severe cases or when NSAIDs are not suitable, corticosteroids may be used to reduce inflammation.

Medications to Improve Uric Acid Excretion:

• **Probenecid:** This medication helps increase the excretion of uric acid by the kidneys. It is often used in cases where there is underexcretion of uric acid.

Supplements:

Vitamin C:

• Some studies suggest that vitamin C supplementation may help lower uric acid levels. Foods rich in vitamin C, such as citrus fruits and berries, may also be beneficial.

Fish Oil (Omega-3 Fatty Acids):

• Omega-3 fatty acids found in fish oil may have anti-inflammatory properties and could potentially be beneficial for individuals with gout. However, evidence is not conclusive, and consultation with a healthcare professional is advised.

Baking Soda:

• Baking soda (sodium bicarbonate) may be used as an adjunct to other treatments to alkalinize the urine and increase the solubility of uric acid. However, its use requires careful monitoring due to potential side effects.

Cherry Extract or Cherry Juice:

• Some studies suggest that cherries or cherry extract may help reduce gout attacks. This is believed to be related to their anti-inflammatory properties. However, more research is needed.

It is essential to emphasize that supplements and medications should be used under the guidance of healthcare professionals. Partaking in self-prescribing or self-medicating can lead to adverse outcomes and drug interactions. Enhancing lifestyle through dietary changes and maintaining a healthy weight is crucial for managing disorders related to purine. Always consult a healthcare professional to determine the most appropriate and effective course of treatment based on your specific health condition.

Conclusion

Regulating purine levels is crucial for those with conditions such as gout, kidney stones, or other associated health issues. A comprehensive approach that includes dietary modifications, lifestyle changes, and, if needed, medications and supplements can effectively promote optimal health. Essential points:

Dietary Considerations:

• Adhering to a low purine diet requires selecting foods with reduced purine content and restricting high-purine items including organ meats, specific shellfish, and processed meats.

It is crucial to incorporate lean protein sources, complete grains, and a variety of fruits and vegetables into your diet for balance and nutrition.

• Lifestyle Changes: Ensuring adequate hydration is essential for facilitating the elimination of uric acid via the kidneys.

• Maintaining a healthy weight through regular exercise and a balanced diet can improve overall health and assist in managing purine levels.

• **Medications and Supplements:** - Allopurinol and febuxostat are used to reduce uric acid levels in persons with gout or hyperuricemia.

Anti-inflammatory medications such as NSAIDs or colchicine can help alleviate pain during gout flare-ups.

• Supplements like vitamin C or fish oil may offer advantages, but it is advisable to see a healthcare practitioner before using them.

• **Personalized Approach:** Individual responses to nutritional and medicinal interventions can differ, necessitating personalized guidance from healthcare specialists such as registered dietitians and physicians.

Regularly monitoring uric acid levels and overall health is crucial for optimal management.

• Utilizing a holistic health approach involves integrating dietary adjustments, lifestyle changes, and suitable medical treatments to effectively address purine-related illnesses.

• Considering stress management, sleep quality, and overall well-being adds to a comprehensive and enduring approach to health.

Successful treatment of purine levels necessitates a cooperative approach involving patients and their healthcare team. Individuals may make informed decisions and seek professional advice to improve and sustain their optimal health. Consistent communication with healthcare providers enables continuous assessment and modifications to the management plan as necessary.

THE END